Legal Notice

Disclaimer Notice

Please note the information contained within this document is for educational and entertainment purposes only. Considerable energy and every attempt has been made to provide the most up to date, accurate, relative, reliable, and complete information, but the reader is strongly encouraged to seek professional advice prior to using any of this information contained in this book. The reader understands they are reading and using this information contained herein at their own risk, and in no way will the author, publisher, or any affiliates be held responsible for any damages whatsoever. No warranties of any kind are expressed or implied. Readers acknowledge that the author is not engaging in the rendering of legal, financial, medical, or any other professional advice. By reading this document, the reader agrees that under no circumstances is the author, publisher, or anyone else affiliated with the production, distribution, sale, or any other element of this book responsible for any losses, direct or indirect, which are incurred as a result of the use of information contained within this document, including, but not limited to, -errors, omissions, or inaccuracies. Because of the rate with which conditions change, the author and publisher reserve the right to alter and update the information contained herein on the new conditions whenever they see applicable.

Table Of Contents

Ultimate Fast Metabolism Recipe Cookbook!

Fast Metabolism

Metabolism Boosting Paleo Recipes, Low Carb Recipes, Gluten Free Recipes, And Detox Smoothies To Get In Shape And Lose Weight Fast!

Sarah Brooks

STOP!!! Before you read any further....Would you like to know the Secrets of Body Transformation?

If your answer is yes, then you are not alone. Thousands of people are looking for the secret to rapidly burn body fat, keep the weight off, become healthier, and truly transform their body and life for good.

If you have been searching for these answers without much luck, you are in the right place!

Not only will you gain incredible insight in this book, but because I want to make sure to give you as much value as possible, right now for a limited time you can get full **100% FREE access to a VIP bonus EBook** entitled **THE 7 KEYS TO BODY TRANSFORMATION!**

Introduction

I want to thank you and congratulate you for purchasing the book, **Fast Metabolism: Ultimate Fast Metabolism Recipe Cookbook! Metabolism Boosting Paleo Recipes, Low Carb Recipes, Gluten Free Recipes, And Detox Smoothies To Get In Shape And Lose Weight Fast!**

This book contains proven steps and strategies on how to lose weight effectively by increasing your metabolism through proper diet.

Losing weight is not an easy thing to do. Some people have given up because they feel that their efforts are put into waste. But the real problem is the way you consume your foods. Although your aim is to shed off your extra pounds, it doesn't mean you have to starve yourself and eat lesser and lesser.

In this book, you will learn the effective way of losing weight through diets such as:

- Paleo Diet
- Low-carb Diet
- Gluten-free Diet
- Detox Smoothies

Also included in this book are some delicious and nutritious recipes that you will surely love. These recipes will not only increase your energy but will also boost your metabolism.

Thanks again for purchasing this book, I hope you enjoy it!

Chapter 1: Why Do Some People Have Faster Metabolisms Than Others, And How Can You Make Yours Faster?

To put it simply, metabolism is the function in the body wherein the foods that you consume are processed into energy. This process is actually the combination of catabolism and anabolism. Catabolism is when your body breaks down food and turns them into energy. Anabolism is when the body uses those nutrients to rebuild itself and store the extra as body fat.

Energy consumption of the body is divided into three main metabolic rates:

- Resting Metabolic Rate (RMR) – this is the energy used by your body to keep your organs working (heart pumping, lungs breathing, etc.) while you are resting or asleep. Basal Metabolic Rate basically measures the same thing but the standards used for quantifying are stricter and are more ideal for lab research.
- Activity-induced thermogenesis – The energy you need to do your daily activities such as walking, running, washing the dishes, cleaning the house, exercise, etc. In short, this is the energy you need to accomplish things aside from lying down or sitting.
- Thermic effect of food or diet-induced thermogenesis – this is the energy needed to be able to break down the foods that you eat and absorb their nutrients.

Since the energy in the body is used in these three main areas, the metabolism of each individual differs on how the energy is distributed among these three. Some people burns more calories during exercise, others burn more calories from breaking down the foods that they consume while others have a faster RMR. RMR varies with gender, age, race and level of fitness. Genes and food intake also affects metabolism.

When you starve yourself in the hope of losing more fats, it can cause your metabolism to slow down in response because your body is required to conserve more energy to keep you alive. Eating more can raise your metabolism but it is not enough to burn the extra calories you have consumed. The role of genes in metabolism is not clear. Although you cannot deny that genes play a role in metabolism, it is not the only factor and it does not necessarily mean that you will be obese forever just because of genetically slow metabolism.

Activity-induced thermogenesis or the amount of energy required for more energy-consuming, voluntary activities such as exercise is the easiest to change and control since it depends on how much physical activities you do. You can choose to do sprinting that burns more calories or choose to walk instead and burn lesser calories. You are in control of what physical activity you would perform on a day to day basis. Your choice of activity differs from the others, therefore, the amount of calories you burn vary from the amount of calories that others are able to burn.

Diet-induced thermogenesis requires the least calories to burn the foods that you consume and absorb the nutrients they contain. It is affected by various factors such as:

- Macronutrient composition of the food that you consume
- Temperature of the food
- Size of your meal
- Chemical contained in the food itself

It is now clear that metabolism is affected by many factors but, is there a way for you to make yours faster? The answer is yes. From the factors outlined above, it is clear that something can be done about slow metabolism.

Build lean muscles. For women, you do not have to worry about getting huge muscles since this is only achieved by lifting very heavy weights and taking unnatural supplements. You can build lean muscles by having the right diet and having an exercise routine that works best for your body. Having more muscles in your body will help burn calories. During workout, your metabolism increases since you need more energy to perform the exercise routines. Additionally, your RMR will also increase because your body needs more calories to repair your muscle tissues while you are at rest.

Cardiovascular exercise. You need to alternately perform a high intensity workout and a low intensity workout incorporated in your exercise routine. For example, run for 2 minutes then fast run for 30 seconds and do a sprint. Repeat the routine for 20 minutes. You can choose whatever workout you like best as long as it alternates between high and low intensity. Doing so will not only increase your metabolism but your RMR as well. This is because your heart pumps faster and it needs more energy to keep pumping harder, therefore burning more calories.

Eat frequently with smaller amounts. A lot of people are misled with this idea. It is true that eating more each day increases your metabolic rate but if you eat too much, your increased metabolism will not be enough to burn all the calories you have consumed, therefore, the excess will be stored as fats. The idea here is to keep your digestive system active and prevent hunger pangs and food cravings. The proper way to do this is to eat at least 4 to 6 small meals each day. You don't have to be very full each meal as this will result to overeating. As long as you are able to put food in your stomach and you are no longer hungry, (not necessarily full) it should be enough.

Add healthy fats in your diet. Omega 3 fatty acids, monounsaturated fats and other healthy fats should be included in your diet. These healthy fats aid in proper metabolism. Omega 3 fatty acid helps regulate blood sugar level, reduces risk of inflammation and decreases your vulnerability to leptin (protein that regulates the fat storage in the body).

Drink green tea. Green tea contains Catechins which is a thermogenic and has been proven to reduce body fat when consumed daily at a certain amount. According to a clinical study published in The American Journal of Clinical Nutrition, drinking tea with 690mg of Catechins for 12 weeks reduce body fats. This suggests that consumption of green tea can help improve and prevent diseases such obesity and other life-style related diseases.

Avoid drastically lowering your calories. When you go on a low-calorie diet or do fasting (starvation) diet, your metabolism will slow down in the long run. When the amount of calorie in your body is very low, your body will think that you are starving. Therefore, your body will minimize fat loss in order to keep your energy level to normal. You can safely lower down your calorie intake by having more meals each day. Just make sure that your meals are in smaller portions, around 300 calories per meal should suffice.

Start your day right by having proper breakfast. Eat good foods during breakfast to help you sustain your level of energy for the day. Eat foods rich in protein and carbohydrates. Eating proper breakfast also helps increase your metabolism. This is because when you eat breakfast, you prevent yourself from starvation eating later in the day wherein you tend to eat more because you feel so hungry, you binge mindlessly. When you eat breakfast, your body is fueled so your body does not feel starved during lunch and dinner, you don't overeat. This way, you are able to distribute the calories in your body throughout the day.

Trans Fat is a big NO! Trans-fatty acids are industrially-processed hydrogen that is added to liquid vegetable oils to give them a more solid texture, thus the term "partially hydrogenated oils'. Trans Fat raises LDL or bad cholesterol and lowers down HDL or good cholesterol in the body. This can result to cardiovascular diseases and increases the risk for Type 2 Diabetes. Eat fresh fruits and vegetables instead. They are not only healthy; they also taste great and help in better metabolism. Grapefruit, for example, helps boost your metabolism by lowering down your insulin level. Apples help curb food cravings and enhance digestion while berries boost your fat-burning abilities and helps improve your overall health.

Stay away from low-fat, low-carb, sugar-free foods that claims to be healthy foods. These foods may have lower carbohydrates or lower fats but chances are other bad components are increased or are used to replace the other one. They can use aspartame instead or add more sugar or other chemicals to compensate for the other one. So they are not healthy after all and you are just putting your health at risk.

Eat more green vegetables. The darker they are the better. Dark green vegetables contain more fiber which boosts the digestive system resulting to better absorption of nutrients from food. They are also rich in iron which supports the red blood cells for better transport of nutrients in the entire body.

Spice it up! Adding hot spices to your food such as chili peppers, cayenne and jalapeño will help increase your fat burning abilities because they contain Capsaicin. Capsaicin helps increase the fat-burning hormones in your body.

Avoid eating late at night. When you eat late at night, your body will not be able to process all the calories that you have consumed since your body is at rest when it is sleeping. Therefore, those calories that you consumed are stored as fats and slow down your metabolism.

Get enough sleep. It has been proven that sleeping 7 to 8 hours a day helps improve your brain functions, your energy levels and your metabolism.

Stay away from stress. When you are stressed, Cortisol is released in your body and too much of it is stored as fats. Relieve your stress by doing some simple exercises, do your hobbies, eat more fresh fruits and laugh a lot.

Chapter 2: Advantages Of The Paleo Diet And Increasing Metabolism

Paleo Diet allows you to eat foods without the need to count their calorie-content. Since Paleo Diet concentrates on eating lean meats, whole, unprocessed foods and organic fruits and vegetables, it is easy to see that it is a healthy diet that can help increase your metabolism. Going on a Paleo diet means no refined sugar or grains, the main causes of insulin-resistance in the body. Furthermore, by eating natural, organic foods, you are preventing yourself from being subjected to harmful chemicals that are added in processed foods.

Unlike other diets out there, you will not starve with Paleo. In fact, you are allowed to eat 4 to 6 times each day in smaller meals. The Paleo Diet is also packed with protein-rich foods which help increase your metabolism. Organic fruits are also rich in fiber and nutrients that help reduce insulin-resistance which leads to better metabolism. Green leafy vegetables are rich in fiber which supports better digestion. This means your body gets healthier since it is able to absorb the food nutrients effectively.

Furthermore, Paleo diet requires you to move your body or have a regular exercise routine to help shed off extra fats. You also get to have enough sleep regularly with this diet which is crucial if you want to lose weight effectively and faster.

Chapter 3: Delicious Fast Metabolism Paleo Recipes

Paleo Crab Cakes

Ingredients:

1lb fresh lump crab meat

1 large egg

2 tablespoons Paleo mayonnaise

1 teaspoon Dijon mustard

¼ teaspoon hot pepper sauce

¼ teaspoon lemon juice

½ teaspoon Worcestershire sauce

¼ cup and 1/3 cup almond flour

2 teaspoon green onions, sliced

1 tablespoon red pepper, finely diced

1 tablespoon fresh parsley, chopped

Directions:

Grease a baking sheet. In a mixing bowl, whisk the egg, Dijon mustard, Paleo mayonnaise, Worcestershire sauce, lemon juice, hot sauce and black pepper. Whisk until ingredients are well blended.

Place the crab meat in another mixing bowl and add the egg mixture that you just whisked. Gently combine ingredients using your hands. Add ¼ cup almond flour, green onions, peppers and freshly chopped parsley. Thus mixture is good for 6 patties.

In a shallow bowl, place the other cup of almond flour and use it to dredge the patties. Arrange the patties in the greased baking sheet and leave in the refrigerator for 1 hour.

Preheat oven to 200°C (400°F) and bake the patties for 15 to 20 minutes or until they are golden brown.

Beefy Vegetable Sautee

Ingredients

½ kilo lean grass-fed beef meat (cut into 1 inch long strips)

1 medium head cabbage, cut into strips

1 large carrot, julienned

2 tablespoon onion leeks (cut into thin, diagonal strips)

2 cloves garlic, crushed and minced

2 medium sweet potatoes (peeled and cut into thin strips)

½ teaspoon Worcestershire sauce

½ teaspoon sea salt

Ground pepper to taste

2 tablespoon coconut oil

½ cup water

In a cooking pan, heat the coconut oil in medium fire. Sautee garlic until it starts to smell. Add the beef meat and sauté until meat is no longer red. Add water. Simmer until tender. Add sweet potatoes and mix. Toss in the carrots, mix and cover for 2 minutes. Add the Worcestershire sauce and ground pepper. Mix in cabbage strips and season with sea salt. Mix and cover for a minute. Turn off heat and serve.

Healthy Breakfast Omelet

Ingredients:

3 large free-range eggs

Ground black pepper

Fresh basil leaves (finely chopped)

Sea salt

2 tablespoons coconut oil

2 tablespoon coconut cream

1 small onion, julienned

2 cloves garlic (crushed and minced)

Whisk the eggs in a mixing bowl and add coconut cream and sea salt. Heat the cooking pan in medium heat and add coconut oil. When hot, sauté garlic and onion. Pour the egg mixture and while it's still syrupy, sprinkle top with finely chopped basil leaves. When the sides are already solid, roll one side going to the other side. Flip it over. Turn off heat but leave the egg to cook some more. Remove from pan and serve with brown rice and soup.

Ultimate Chicken Wings

Ingredients:

1 kilo free-range chicken wings

4 clove garlic, crushed and minced

1 small red onion, minced

2 large red chili peppers

Finely ground black pepper

1 teaspoon ground cumin

1 teaspoon sea salt

½ cup fresh cilantro leaves

1 lemon (juiced)

Blend all the ingredients together, except for the chicken wings. Blend until the mixture is smooth and pour into a zip lock bag. Add in the chicken wings and toss until the chicken wings are fully covered with the blended marinade. Leave in the refrigerator overnight.

Preheat your oven to 200°C. Cover your baking tray with foil and arrange the chicken wings. Bake each side for 15 minutes or until brown. You may serve as is or serve with a dip.

Green Leafy Bacon Salad

Ingredients:

1 pound nitrate-free bacon

1 medium head Romaine lettuce

1 small white onion, julienned

1 teaspoon honey

1 large tomato, cut into round, thin slices

1 teaspoon lemon juice

Sea salt

Finely ground black pepper

In a non-stick pan, heat the bacon slice until they become crispy. Cool and chop into smaller bits. Set aside.

In a big salad bowl, arrange the Romaine lettuce. Cut the leaves using your hands. In a small bowl, mix together the rest of the ingredients until well combined. Pour mixture on top of the Romaine lettuce. Sprinkle with bacon bits. Cool and serve.

Chapter 4: Advantages Of The Low Carb Diet And Increasing Metabolism

The Paleo Diet, Gluten-free Diet and Low Carb Diet has one thing in common, they all involve eating natural, unprocessed foods. Of course, they have differences, but you can't deny the fact that the best way to lose weight and increase your metabolism is by eating natural foods.

Low Carb Diet is basically eating natural foods that contain low carbohydrates. For some, the Low Carb Diet is the best diet for those who want to lose weight, optimize their health and lower their risk of having diseases. For those who are suffering from insulin resistance, the Low Carb Diet is an advantage because it lowers down the basal insulin levels and blood glucose, factors which affect normal body metabolism.

For any diet, you do not have to starve yourself. For the Low Carb Diet, you just need to remember the basics: eat fruits, vegetables and non-gluten grains (in moderation) and do not eat sugar, wheat, Trans fat, artificial sweeteners, processed foods and low-fat products.

Natural, low-carb foods include meat, fish, eggs, vegetables, fruits, nuts, seeds, high-fat dairy, fats and oils.

Meat – Any poultry animals will do but grass-fed is better.

Fish – Any fish will do but opt for wild-caught if available.

Vegetables – Cauliflower, carrots, broccoli, spinach and other green leafy veggies.

Fruits – Oranges, pears, apples, strawberries and blueberries are best.

Nuts and seeds – Sunflower seeds, walnuts, almonds and others.

High-fat dairy – Heavy cream, yogurt, butter and cheese.

Fats and oils – Olive oil, cod fish liver oil, lard, butter and coconut oil.

You may also eat organic dark chocolate with 70% cocoa but only in moderation especially if you are trying to lose weight.

Chapter 5: Delicious Fast Metabolism Low Carb Recipes

Mini Broccoli and Cheese Egg Cakes

Ingredients:

4 large eggs

1 cup egg whites

4 cups broccoli florets

¼ cup shredded cheddar

¼ cup grated cheese

1 teaspoon olive oil

Salt

Ground black pepper

Preheat your oven to 350°F. Use a bit of water to steam the broccoli florets for about 6 to 7 minutes. When the broccoli is done, crumble them into smaller pieces in a bowl and mix with salt, pepper and olive oil.

Beat the egg whites, eggs, grated cheese, ground pepper and salt. Grease your standard non-stick muffin tray and pour the mixture over each tin until ¾ full. Top each tin with grated cheddar and bake for 20 minutes or until cooked. Serve while hot.

You can store your leftovers in a plastic wrap and keep in the refrigerator for a few days. You can microwave the leftovers and serve while hot.

Bacon-wrapped Ground Beef

Ingredients:

8 strips of bacon

½ lb bacon cut into small chunks

1 lb ground beef

¼ cup coconut milk

1/3 cup fresh chives, minced

2 garlic cloves, minced

Finely ground black pepper

Salt to taste

Preheat oven to 400°F. Mix together the ground beef, bacon chunks, coconut milk, chives and black pepper. Mix until all the ingredients are well blended and hold together. Grease a regular-sized muffin tin and put a slice of bacon on each side of the hole. Fill each muffin hole with the beef mixture. Bake for 30 minutes.

Cool until you can hold the handle. Remove each bacon-wrapped beef filling from the muffin tray and sprinkle each with chopped parsley on top.

Baked Salmon in Herbs

Ingredients:

2 6oz salmon fillets

1 tablespoon coconut flour

1 tablespoon olive oil

1 tablespoon Dijon mustard

2 tablespoon parsley (fresh or dried)

Salt

Ground black pepper

For the salad:

2 cups arugula

1 lemon (juiced)

1 tablespoon olive oil

1 tablespoon white wine vinegar

½ small red onion, sliced thinly

Salt

Ground pepper

Preheat oven to 450°F. Line your baking sheet with foil and place salmon fillets. Mix together the olive oil and Dijon mustard and rub into the salmon fillets. Set aside. Combine coconut flour, parsley, pepper and salt. Sprinkle the mixture on the salmon fillets using a spoon and pat them onto your hands.

Cook in the oven for 10 to 15 minutes depending on your preference. Meanwhile, mix together all the salad ingredients in a salad bowl. Place the cooked salmon fillets on top of the salad and serve.

Easy Carrot Snack

Ingredients:

A pound of fresh baby carrots

A tablespoon of olive oil

Half teaspoon of salt

Line your baking sheet with foil to avoid heavy scrubbing later. Place the baby carrots in the baking sheet and drizzle with olive oil and salt. Roast for 12 minutes at 475°. Mix and roast again for another 4 minutes. Mix one more time and continue to roast for 4 to 7 minutes or until the carrots become brown and tender. Serve while hot. You can keep your leftovers in tightly sealed plastic bags and store in the refrigerator.

Chapter 6: Advantages Of Gluten Free Eating And Metabolism

Gluten is the combination of two proteins, glutenin and gliadin. Gluten is what gives the dough its elastic texture which keeps it together. In the past, experts thought Celiac disease and gluten intolerance were just isolated cases. It turns out that more and more people are affected by these conditions. Gluten causes vomiting, nauseas, headache, diarrhea, bloating and gas to those who suffer from Celiac disease and Gluten intolerance.

Gluten is mainly found in grains such as rye, barley, wheat, cereals and triticale. If you suffer from Celiac Disease or gluten intolerance, you will benefit from this diet. But just because a product is labeled as "gluten-free" does not mean it is healthier. More often than not, they contain more carbohydrates, calories or fats.

There are a few advantages when you go gluten-free. A gluten-free diet means you will stay away from grains. Since fried foods mostly require breading, you will also cut down your consumption of fried foods. Most desserts are made with flour which comes from wheat or other grains. This means you will also stop consuming sugar-filled and fat-filled desserts and foods.

When you cut down your consumption of sugar, you also lower down your risk to insulin resistance that can lead to Type II Diabetes. Furthermore, you will be forced to eat natural foods such as fruits and vegetables since they contain less starch and gluten-free as well. By eating more natural foods, your body becomes more nutritious and your risk of heart disease, cancer, diabetes and gluten-intolerance are reduced. Since most fruits and vegetables are antioxidants, your body develops higher immunity that prevents many germs and viruses.

It is always better to use natural products to ensure that you get the best. As mentioned above, not all "gluten-free" products available in the market are healthy. You may use brown rice, quinoa or sweet potatoes as substitute for starches since they are gluten-free. By consuming all-natural, nutritious products, you keep your body healthy and boost your metabolism which leads to proper weight loss.

Chapter 7: Delicious Fast Metabolism Gluten Free Recipes

Grilled Steak

Ingredients:

3 pounds beef flank or skirt

Loosely ground black pepper

1/3 cup lime juice

½ cup cumin seeds

5 pieces chopped Jalapeño peppers (seeds and ribs removed)

3 cloves garlic, crushed and minced

1 teaspoon salt

1 teaspoon soy sauce

1 ½ cups olive oil

Cilantro leaves with stem

In a pan, toast the cumin seeds in medium heat until it becomes fragrant. Combine the jalapeños, cumin seeds, garlic, black pepper, salt and lime juice in a blender and blend until ingredients are finely chopped. Add cilantro and olive oil. Blend until mixture becomes smooth as puree.

For the marinade to penetrate into the meat, score each side lightly with a knife. Place the meat in a bowl and pour in the marinade. Make sure to coat all of the meat. Leave in the refrigerator for a day.

Preheat the grill and lightly grease with oil. Grill each side for 2 minutes on high and discard remaining marinade. Turn the heat to low and cook for another 3 to 4 minutes or until your desired doneness. Serve while hot with brown rice or quinoa.

Pork Tenderloin with Quinoa

Ingredients:

1 lb pork tenderloin

¼ cup uncooked quinoa

1 small apple, peeled, cored and chopped

½ onion, chopped

2 cloves garlic, chopped

¼ cup raisins

4 pieces button mushrooms, chopped

2 tablespoons pine nuts

2 tablespoons white wine

2 tablespoons olive oil

A pinch of ground cinnamon

A pinch of salt

A pinch of finely ground black pepper

Garam masala to taste

Boil the quinoa and water in a saucepan over medium heat for about 15 minutes or until the quinoa is tender and the water is fully absorbed. In a skillet, heat the olive oil and sauté the onion, garlic, apples, pine nuts, mushrooms and raisins for about 8 minutes or until the onion turns translucent. Mix in the wine and cook more until the liquid evaporates. Pour the apple mixture into the boiled quinoa and mix until well blended. Set aside.

Preheat your oven to 220°C or 425°F. Cut the pork tenderloin starting from the side going to the middle, just like a widespread book. Pound the cut pork tenderloin using a meat mallet to ½ inch thick. Rub both sides of the pork tenderloin with cinnamon, salt, black pepper and garam masala. Fill the pork tenderloin with the quinoa-apple filling and roll. Secure the pork filling using a toothpick or kitchen twine on both sides and on the middle.

Roast the pork for about 35 minutes or until the pork is brown. You may use an instant-read thermometer and insert it into the center of the pork. When the temperature reads 145°F or 63°C, the roasted pork is done. Cover it with aluminum foil and leave to rest for 10 minutes. Slice and serve.

Gluten-Free Pancakes

Ingredients:

1 cup rice flour

1/3 cup potato starch

3 tablespoons Tapioca flour

½ teaspoon baking soda

½ teaspoon salt

1 ½ teaspoon baking powder

½ teaspoon Xanthan gum

1 ¾ cup buttermilk

2 tablespoon honey

3 tablespoons applesauce

2 cups water

2 eggs (large)

Sift together the dry ingredients such as baking soda, baking powder, salt, tapioca flour, potato starch and rice flour. Add in the eggs, applesauce, water, honey and xanthan gum. Mix until no lumps are left.

Grease skillet with butter or oil and heat over medium fire. Pour batter onto the skillet. When bubbles start to form on the edges, flip the pancake. Continue cooking until the bottom is brown. You may also add dried fruits into the batter. Serve immediately with some fresh berries on the side.

Chapter 8: When To Use Detox Smoothies And How To Best Use Them To Increase Your Metabolism

Detox smoothies are very easy to prepare and they are undeniably tasty and very nutritious. If you want to lose some weight or you simply want a healthier body, you can add Detox Smoothies to your diet.

Detox smoothies offer many advantages:

- Detoxifying and Alkalizing – this is true with green smoothies since they contain chlorophyll that initiates detox and alkalizes the body to get rid of toxins accumulated from the environment and foods consumed.
- Anti-inflammatory – vegetables and fruits have anti-inflammatory properties that helps prevent diseases such as arthritis and cancer.
- Better digestion – fruits and vegetables are rich in fiber that boosts digestion. Therefore, your body is able to absorb more nutrients since you are able to digest the foods that you eat properly. Better absorption of nutrients help increase metabolism.
- Weight loss – Detox smoothies uses fruits and vegetables that are high in vitamins, minerals and antioxidants. They are also low in fat and sugar that is why detox smoothies support natural weight loss.
- Increased energy – Detox smoothies are full of nutrients and are easily digested by the body. Therefore, the nutrients are easily transported all over the body, leading to better metabolism and increased energy.

If you want to have a healthier body, increase your energy and enhance your body's metabolism, adding Detox Smoothies to your diet is a must.

Chapter 9: Gourmet Detox Smoothies For A Faster Metabolism

Raspberry Ginger Smoothie

This smoothie is great for breakfast as it aids in better digestion and detoxifies the body as well.

Blend 1 cup fresh raspberries (frozen will do but go for the unsweetened one), ¾ cup almond milk or rice milk (chilled), ¼ cup pitted cherries, 2 tablespoons honey, 2 tablespoons finely grated ginger, 1 teaspoon flaxseed (ground) and 1 teaspoon lemon juice. Puree the mixture until smooth. Serve in chilled glasses.

Green Smoothie Delight

This green smoothie does not only taste great, it is also a good way to purge toxins out of your body.

Ingredients:

1 ¼ cup cubed green mangoes

¼ cup fresh mint, chopped

1 ¼ cups Kale leaves (tough ribs and stems removed)

2 medium celery ribs, chopped

¼ cup parsley, chopped

1 cup orange juice (chilled)

Process all ingredients in a blender and blend until smooth. Serve in chilled glasses.

Fruits and Chia Seeds Smoothie

This smoothie is not only satisfying; it is also packed with fiber for better digestion and nutrients for increased energy and better metabolism.

Blend ¼ avocado, ½ pears, and a cup of spinach with ¼ cup coconut water, a cup of almond milk, a teaspoon of chia seeds and ¼ cup water. Puree until desired smoothness and serve.

Papaya Coco Smoothie

Drink to a healthier tummy and faster metabolism.

In a blender, combine a cup of ripe papaya, a cup of coconut kefir (cultured coconut milk or coconut yogurt are other options), freshly squeezed lime juice from ½ lime and 1 teaspoon honey. Puree until you get a smooth consistency. Serve in chilled glasses.

Strawberries and Greens Smoothie

This smoothie is a healthy way to start your day.

In a blender, mix the following:

10 fresh strawberries, leaves removed

1 whole orange, peeled and wedged

1 ½ cups spinach

1 ½ cups kale

1 cup ripe mango

1 cup pineapples, cubed

1/3 Greek yogurt

1 tablespoon honey

¼ cup water

Blend all ingredients until your desired smoothness. Serve in chilled glasses. Enjoy!

Banana Kale Ginger Goodness

Combine 1 cup bananas, 1 cup blueberries, 1 cup chopped Kale, 1 tablespoon chopped ginger, 1 tablespoon chia seeds, 1 tablespoon honey and 1 cup almond milk in a blender. Puree until smooth.

This Detox smoothie is very refreshing and will keep you feeling satisfied for a while.

Conclusion

Thank you again for purchasing this book on how to increase your metabolism through proper diet!

I am extremely excited to pass this information along to you, and I am so happy that you now have read and can hopefully implement these strategies going forward.

I hope this book was able to help you understand how metabolism works and how to increase your metabolism naturally. By following the diets discussed in this book, you are surely on your way to a healthier, fitter and stronger body.

The next step is to get started using this information and to hopefully live a disease-free, happier and fulfilled life!

Please don't be someone who just reads this information and doesn't apply it, the strategies in this book will only benefit you if you use them!

If you know of anyone else that could benefit from the information presented here please inform them of this book.

Finally, if you enjoyed this book and feel it has added value to your life in any way, please take the time to share your thoughts and post a review on Amazon. It'd be greatly appreciated!

Thank you and good luck!

Preview Of:

Mindfulness Meditation Guide To:

Feeling Good

Relieve Stress, Stop Worrying, Develop Self Confidence And Trust, And Live In The Moment!

Introduction

I want to thank you and congratulate you for purchasing the book, *"Feeling Good: Mindfulness Meditation Guide To Feeling Good! - Relieve Stress, Stop Worrying, Develop Self Confidence And Trust, And Live In The Moment!"*.

Feeling Good And Living In The Present Moment Is Easier Than It Seems!

Whether you are a beginner at meditation or more advanced, "Feeling Good" contains proven steps and strategies on how to use mindfulness meditations and relaxation techniques to have you take your level of consciousness to the next level.

It is truly surprising to me how many people live in an anxious, worried, and overall unhappy state on an everyday basis. Maybe you are one of these unfortunate people who have somehow gotten yourself in a perpetual state of not feeling good. Or maybe you occasionally are feeling good, but often times you feel bad. No matter your circumstance this book is here to provide quick, concise, accurate, and easy to implement strategies to get you in the feeling good state and winning in life!

The book will guide you through understanding what mindfulness is and how to become mindful by practicing meditation. It also contains effective meditation techniques to make you feel good and truly live in the moment, given in easy step by step details. You also get to incorporate mindfulness meditation in your everyday life in by following a simple routine. Lastly, you will learn the small but highly beneficial habits that will help you to live and enjoy the present moment.

Thanks again for purchasing this book, I hope you enjoy it!

Chapter 1 - Mindfulness And Feeling Good

When we start to pay attention to the present moment, we become more aware of ourselves and our life. The past is forever gone and the future is a complete blank. The present moment, the experience and the surroundings that you have right here and now, is what you really have. This sense of awareness is called mindfulness.

What mindfulness really is?

Simply put, mindfulness came from the ancient Indian word "satt", which means awareness, attention and remembering. You become aware of the present moment; you pay attention to your awareness of the present moment; and you remember to pay attention to each experience from each moment.

When you put mindfulness into action, you pay attention to something or someone in particular. You become aware of the way things are right now, not what they were or will be. However, you do not react to it; you respond. Reaction is when you do something automatically without thinking. Response is when you become more mindful and reflective as you take action.

By being mindful, you are also being non-judgmental. Most of us judge an experience in black or white, good or bad. By becoming non-judgmental, your mind's eye is not clouded by your opinions based on your past. Instead, you begin to perceive things as they are now.

Lastly, being mindful means being openhearted. In anything and everything, you bring with you the elements of warmth, kindness and compassion.

How do you start becoming mindful?

One way to become mindful is to do mindfulness meditation. This involves focusing your attention in a systematic way to whatever it is that you decide to concentrate on. This includes the awareness of your thoughts. You become more aware of the repeated patterns that your thoughts make once you take the time to listen to them.

These patterns have a major effect on how you feel and the decisions that you make at the present moment.

Why it's important to live in the present moment and feel good?

People sometimes get lost in their thoughts, and sometimes these thoughts are harmful for you. For instance, you go on vacation at a relaxing beach to calm your mind, but your mind is deep in thoughts regarding your responsibilities at work. This prevents you from living in the present moment and triggers feelings such as anxiety, depression or stress, all of which keep you from feeling good.

The present moment is all that we really have. Sadly, most of us do not focus on it; instead, we focus too much on the past or the future. We make our present moment run on autopilot. A person who is lost in his thoughts does not feel the sand under his feet nor the cool breeze against his cheek. He does not get to experience feeling good from these because his mind is too focused on regrets from the past or worries over the future.
But you can change that, right now. Mindfulness helps you heal from stress, regret, pain and depression. It will boost your creativity and energy. Ultimately, you start to feel good.

The first step to mindfulness is to meditate, and the next chapter will be your guide.

Thanks for Previewing My Exciting Book Entitled:

"Feeling Good: Mindfulness Meditation Guide To: Relieve Stress, Stop Worrying, Develop Self Confidence And Trust, And Live In The Moment!"

To purchase this book, simply go to the Amazon Kindle store and simply search:

"FEELING GOOD"

Then just scroll down until you see my book. You will know it is mine because you will see my name "Sarah Brooks" underneath the title.

Alternatively, you can visit my author page on Amazon to see this book and other work I have done. Thanks so much, and please don't forget your free bonuses

DON'T LEAVE YET! - CHECK OUT YOUR FREE BONUSES BELOW!

Free Bonus Offer: Get Free Access To The LiveFitVIP.com VIP Newsletter!

Once you enter your email address you will immediately get free access to this awesome newsletter!

But wait, right now if you join now for free you will also get free access to the "The 7 Keys To Body Transformation" free EBook!

To claim both your FREE VIP NEWSLETTER MEMBERSHIP and your FREE BONUS eBook on THE 7 KEYS TO BODY TRANSFORMATION!

Just Go To

www.liveFitVIP.com

www.ingramcontent.com/pod-product-compliance
Lightning Source LLC
Chambersburg PA
CBHW070844290526
45795CB00002B/985
* 9 7 8 1 5 1 4 3 8 1 5 1 9 *